Releasing Verdicts

Path to Peace:

lost to the breeze production

A six-month journey into presence and acceptance.

This journal includes mindfulness prompts and optional physical practices such as stretching, breathwork, grounding, and cold exposure. While these practices are generally safe for most people, please use your best judgment and always consult a qualified healthcare provider before beginning any new physical or mental health routine—especially if you have preexisting conditions.
This journal is not a replacement for medical advice, therapy, or emergency care.

<u>Your well-being is important.</u>

Stay safe, and <u>listen to your body</u>.

For those who would be free

Welcome
to the Path to Peace series

Journaling is one of the most powerful tools we have for understanding ourselves.

When combined with mindfulness, it becomes something even deeper: a practice of meeting each moment with curiosity, compassion, and acceptance.

This series is designed to guide you through six essential aspects of mindfulness.

Begin Again
Approaching each experience as if for the first time

Releasing Verdicts
Letting go of labels and criticism

In the Waiting
Allowing your life to unfold in its own time

Comforting Fall
Believing in your capacity to grow and heal

Space Between
Releasing the constant urge to improve

All That Remains
Embracing yourself and your life as they are

Each of these qualities supports the others.
Together, they create a foundation for greater peace, resilience, and self-understanding.
This is not the only way to practice mindfulness.
It is simply one path among many—
a gentle companion for anyone who wants to walk more kindly with themselves.
You are free to adapt, skip, or revisit any part of this journal.
There is no right or wrong way to begin.
Wherever you start is exactly the right place.

Releasing Verdicts

Welcome to Releasing Verdicts — a 30-day practice of letting go of judgment,
one moment at a time.
This month invites you to observe your thoughts, feelings, and experiences without immediately labeling them as good or bad.
So much of our suffering doesn't come from what happens, but from the stories we attach to what happens.
When we pause, witness, and breathe instead of label and react
we create space.
And in that space, understanding and compassion can begin to grow.
Modern research backs this up:
studies in mindfulness-based stress reduction (MBSR) show that decreasing habitual self-judgment can lead to lower stress levels, improved emotional regulation, and greater resilience. Letting go of blame
— especially toward ourselves —
is one of the most powerful healing shifts we can make.
Over the next 30 days, you'll learn how to notice your automatic reactions without needing to fix, fight, or flee them. Non-judging doesn't mean pretending everything is okay or giving up your voice
it means meeting life with openness instead of verdicts.
And sometimes,
that tiny shift changes everything.

Judgment is a survival reflex. The brain evolved to sort quickly — safe or unsafe, familiar or strange, right or wrong. But while this helped our ancestors avoid danger, it can trap us today in loops of overthinking, shame, and separation. Every time we say "I should be better" or "this is wrong," we reinforce neural grooves that can tighten into anxiety or even self-rejection.

That's why Releasing Verdicts is not just a mindset—it's a somatic process.

Somatics means we practice through the body, not just through ideas.

Judgment often lives as tension: a clenched jaw, a hunched back, a held breath.

When we soften into awareness, we notice where those verdicts live physically—and gently, we begin to loosen them. Breath by breath, we reclaim space inside ourselves.

Philosophically, non-judging invites us to enter each moment like a beginner. Spiritually, it's a radical act of presence — choosing to see clearly rather than react unconsciously. To witness without naming is to return to innocence, to possibility, to the part of you that has always been whole.

In this month, you are not asked to be passive. You are invited to be awake.

To feel.

To soften.

To see without the need to define.

Let's begin.

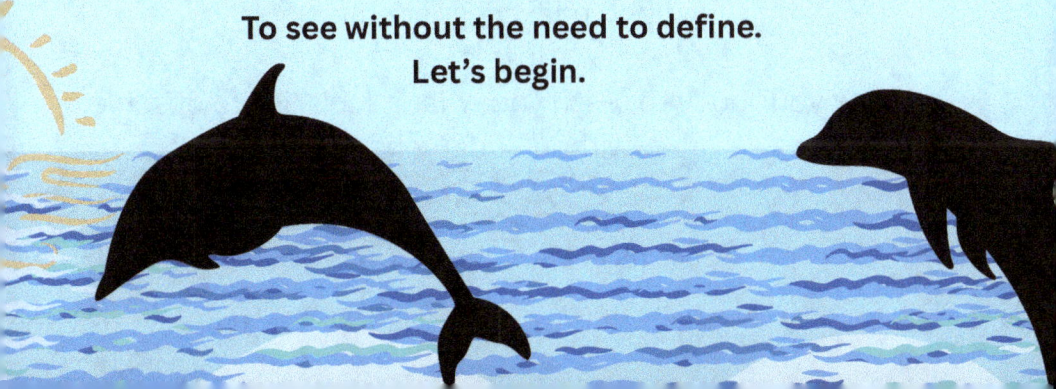

Releasing Verdicts

What are your expectations for this month?

Are you hoping to "get it right," to feel a certain way, or to avoid uncomfortable thoughts?
Take a moment to notice your expectations
about the practice, about yourself, or about what progress should look like.
Can you greet those expectations without judgment? What might shift if you could loosen your grip on them?

Letting go of expectations isn't about abandoning hope—it's about softening your grip on how things should unfold so you can meet them as they are.
Psychologically, unexamined expectations often create the very tension that mindfulness seeks to ease. By noticing them gently, you begin cultivating a practice of awareness without evaluation
A cornerstone of realeasing judgements.

Daily activity

"I'm not detecting any hostile intent..."

Today use your awareness to conduct a body scan. As you move through each part of your body, simply notice without labeling
tight, relaxed, good, bad
just is.
Allow your body to teach you what it feels like to observe without judgment.

Let this month unravel gently
no urgency, no judgment.

Date: _____

Releasing Verdicts

What situations trigger the strongest judgments in you? Why do you think that is?

Think of the moments that provoke instant reactions
whether directed at yourself or others.
Is it when someone drives poorly?
When you feel ignored, criticized, or out of control?
Beneath that spike of judgment, what lives there?
Often, it's something deeper:
a wound, a fear, a need to feel safe.
This isn't about excusing the behavior or dismissing your reaction.
It's about meeting the why without tightening around it.
Can you simply notice the surge of judgment as a messenger?
Not a moral failing?

Daily activity

"Dismiss the Jury"
Close your eyes and imagine an internal courtroom.
You're on trial before a jury of your past voices and inner critics. One by one, breathe out their judgment and mentally dismiss them.
Finally, dissolve the entire courtroom.
Let silence remain. Ask gently:

"Without judgment, what remains?"

A harsh thought is rarely the root
It is the echo of something buried

Date: _____

Releasing Verdicts

When you judge yourself harshly, whose voice does it sound like?

Is it truly yours?
or someone else's, past or present?
Where did that tone begin, and why has it lingered?
Often, the inner critic borrows its voice from those who once had power over us:
a parent, a teacher, a culture, a comment long past.
Over time, that voice we absorbed becomes mistaken for our own.
Today, gently trace the echo. Who are you still carrying and do they truly belong in your self-talk?

Daily activity

Who's in There?

Psychologists call it "introjection" when we unconsciously internalize external judgments.
Today, write a short letter to your inner critic, giving it the name or voice it reminds you of. Don't aim to fight or shame it. Instead, thank it for its effort to protect you, then kindly let it know:
You're not needed in that role anymore.
When you're done, step outside.
Take three slow, mindful breaths and stretch your arms open to the sky. Let that physical openness signal your readiness to release what was never truly yours.
Studies show that open-body postures can reduce cortisol and increase confidence—body leading mind into freedom.

We inherit many voices.
Peace begins when we remember they aren't ours.

Date: _____

Releasing Verdicts

When a strong emotion rises —sadness, anger, fear— what do you do first?

Do you welcome it, resist it, hide it, or try to fix it?
What do you think taught you to respond that way?
We often inherit emotional responses the way we inherit language. Quietly, through observation and repetition.
Maybe you were praised for composure, or scolded for crying.
Maybe survival meant staying calm, staying quiet, staying useful. But emotions are messages, not threats.
Research in affective neuroscience suggests that suppressing emotions can heighten stress, while naming and allowing them can reduce their intensity. So today, just notice your reflex. You don't need to change it—only see it clearly.

Daily activity

Gentle sway and a little hey

When a strong emotion arises today, pause and silently name it—"This is anger," "This is grief," "This is fear." Studies show that this simple act of affect labeling can shift activity from the amygdala to the prefrontal cortex,
reducing reactivity and increasing clarity.
Then, give your body space to process. Stand and slowly sway side to side. Let the emotion move with you, like water rocking in a glass. No urgency to fix—just motion as medicine. Even 60 seconds of gentle movement can ease the nervous system into a more receptive state.

You are not the storm
You are the sky through which it passes

Date: _____

Releasing Verdicts

How does judgment show up in your body? Tightness? Heat? Restlessness?

Where does it settle?
Your chest, jaw, shoulders, gut?
Does it arrive as clenching, heaviness, or numbness?
What if, instead of analyzing it, you simply noticed?
Judgment isn't just a thought
it's a reaction the body holds.
The brain registers judgment as threat, triggering tension and stress responses. But awareness interrupts the pattern. By gently noticing how judgment physically moves through you, you begin to soften its hold.

Daily activity

Mirror Movement

Stand before a mirror for one minute. Soften your gaze—not analyzing, not correcting, just observing. As thoughts arise—good or bad—notice them. Don't push them away or pull them close. Let each thought pass like clouds in the glass. See if you can meet your own reflection without deciding what it means. As thoughts of judgement or correcting your posture or smile arise.
Acknowledge they exist
then without acting on them
allow them to pass.

Judgment settles in the flesh
long before it speaks in the mind

Date: _____

Releasing Verdicts

What would it feel like to witness your thoughts without needing to believe or resist them?

Can you imagine simply noticing what arises?
without labeling it good or bad?
Let each thought drift by like a cloud, neither clung to nor rejected. What space might open if you stopped wrestling with your mind?

Neuroscience shows that mindful awareness of thoughts
—without judgment—
reduces emotional reactivity and strengthens cognitive flexibility. This gentle observation invites a deeper relationship with stillness, curiosity, and inner peace.

Daily activity

"Down the River"

Sit quietly in a comfortable position and watch your thoughts while focusing on your breathing. be like a flowing river with each passing thought being a leaf or stick caught in the current. acknowledge its existence, notice its flow but let it pass.
When a thought arises, silently label it:
"thinking," "judging," "remembering"
then return to your breath.
Let the mind move, but stay anchored in witnessing.

Once you let your thoughts pass
You realize you were always the river

Date: _____

Releasing Verdicts

Bring to mind someone you often judge.
What story have you told yourself about who they are?
and what might that story be missing?

What assumptions have you made about their choices, their
tone, their value? Can you imagine what burdens might shape
their actions?
When we judge, we often replace wonder with certainty.
What shifts if you look again?
With curiosity instead of conclusion?
Social neuroscience reveals that perspective-taking softens
the brain's default bias pathways and increases empathy.
Choosing to imagine another's pain doesn't excuse harm.
It opens a door to deeper understanding.

Daily activity

Empathy Expansion

Set a 5 minute timer.
Close your eyes and picture someone you judge.
Now, imagine one fear they may carry.
One unmet need.
One hope.
Let yourself feel how human they might be.
Just like you.

You don't have to agree to understand.
You only have to be willing to look again.

Date: _____

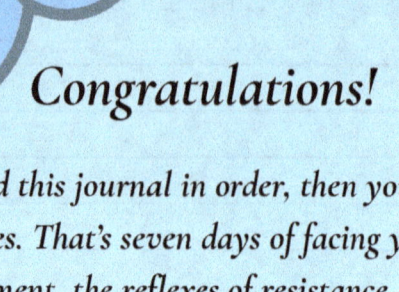

Congratulations!

If you've followed this journal in order, then you've shown up for yourself seven times. That's seven days of facing your inner world — the voices of judgment, the reflexes of resistance, the quiet, complex stories we tell ourselves about ourselves.

Maybe you approached each page with grace.

Maybe some days were heavy, reactive, or messy.

Maybe you skipped a day, then came back anyway.

Whatever your path looked like — I'm proud of you. You showed up not because you had to... but because you chose to. That is a beautiful thing.

Today, I invite you to pause. No prompt. No pressure. No digging or reflecting or rewriting.

Just rest.

Rest your mind.

Relax your body.

Let go of judgment — especially the ones about how you "should" be resting right now.

This is not the end. We're just catching our breath.

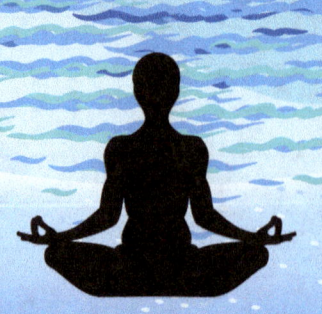

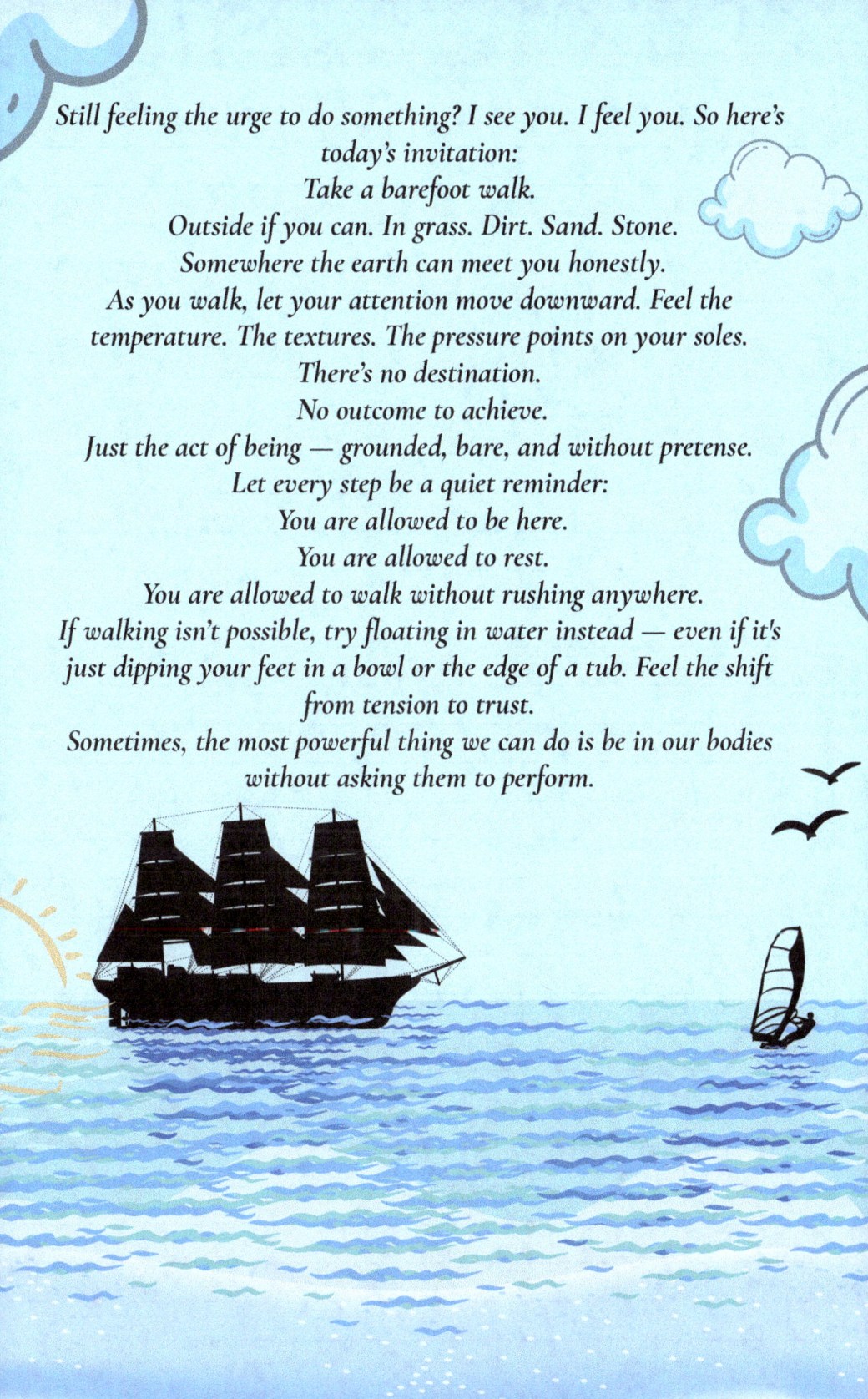

Still feeling the urge to do something? I see you. I feel you. So here's today's invitation:

Take a barefoot walk.

Outside if you can. In grass. Dirt. Sand. Stone.

Somewhere the earth can meet you honestly.

As you walk, let your attention move downward. Feel the temperature. The textures. The pressure points on your soles.

There's no destination.

No outcome to achieve.

Just the act of being — grounded, bare, and without pretense.

Let every step be a quiet reminder:

You are allowed to be here.

You are allowed to rest.

You are allowed to walk without rushing anywhere.

If walking isn't possible, try floating in water instead — even if it's just dipping your feet in a bowl or the edge of a tub. Feel the shift from tension to trust.

Sometimes, the most powerful thing we can do is be in our bodies without asking them to perform.

Date: _____

Date: _____

Releasing Verdicts

Do you think releasing judgements means approving of everything?

Non-judging doesn't ask you to like or agree with what's happening
It asks you to see clearly without hardening into resistance. Judging often triggers tension in the body.
Try this:
When you catch a judgmental thought, pause. Unclench your jaw, lower your shoulders, and take a slow breath. These simple acts can shift your nervous system toward safety, making space for wiser discernment.
Acceptance isn't agreement.
It's the moment you stop arguing with reality long enough to actually understand it.
What happens when you stop labeling an experience and just let it be?

Daily activity

"Nothing to label here"

For five minutes, observe your environment or thoughts without assigning value. A sound is just a sound. A thought, just a thought. If a judgment arises, note it gently ("judging") and return to observing. This simple act helps uncouple awareness from evaluation.

Discernment doesn't require a verdict.
Only presence.

Date: _____

Releasing Verdicts

What role does perfectionism play in your self-judgment?

Does the drive to get it "right" keep you safe?
Or keep you small?
What happens when you fall short of your own expectations?
Explore where perfectionism protects you, where it punishes you, and what might be possible if you let yourself be enough as you are.
Perfectionism often arises from early experiences where approval, safety, or love felt conditional. Over time, it becomes internalized.
A belief that flawlessness equals worth. But studies in self-compassion and mental flexibility show that embracing imperfection fosters resilience and growth, not failure.

Daily activity

Intentional Imperfection:

Choose one task today
—big or small—
Do it imperfectly on purpose.
Let the laundry fold messily, leave the sketch unfinished, write without editing.
As you do, observe the discomfort or freedom that arises.
This is not about sloppiness
It's about softening the grip of judgment.

Perfection is a mask stitched from fear.
It hides your humanity, not your flaws.

Date: _____

Releasing Verdicts

What kinds of people do you tend to judge without realizing it?

Is it strangers on the street? People who speak, dress, or believe differently than you? What quiet stories have you inherited about what's "normal," "right," or "acceptable"? Where did those stories begin, and do they still feel true?

Neuroscience shows our brains naturally sort and categorize it's how we process the world quickly. But those shortcuts can carry unconscious bias, shaped by culture, media, and upbringing.
The antidote isn't guilt
it's awareness.
Curiosity softens reflex, and compassion rehumanizes.

Daily activity

"Where am I?"

Go somewhere you don't usually spend time
a different neighborhood, store, or café. Observe those around you without labeling or explaining. Just notice. If judgment arises, ask yourself: What might this person be facing today? Let the question replace the assumption.

Every person you judge
Is a mirror waiting to be turned inward.

Releasing Verdicts

What happens when you stop deciding if each moment is good or bad, right or wrong?

How does it feel to simply be with experience as it is without needing to fix, label, or resist it? Think of a recent moment when you allowed things to unfold naturally. What did you notice, internally and externally?

Mindfulness research shows that labeling experiences triggers our brain's evaluative networks, narrowing perception. When we pause and simply observe, we engage broader, more receptive awareness. Presence expands. Insight emerges not from control, but from openness.

Daily activity

Learning to Be:

Set a timer for 5 minutes.
Sit quietly and release all goals, responsibilities and burdens
—you can pick them back up when you're done—
As thoughts arise about what's "supposed" to be happening, simply let them go.
Return to the breath, or to the feel of your body in the chair.
Practice being in the moment
no rating, no fixing, no narrative just existing.

Judgment is a habit.
Presence is a choice.

Date: _____

Releasing Verdicts

How might your life feel different if you met more moments with acceptance instead of judgment?

Where do you notice the urge to fix, critique, or control? What happens when that impulse softens, even briefly? Reflect on how more acceptance—of yourself, others, or circumstances—might shift your tone, your tension, or the way you move through the day.
Psychological research suggests that nonjudgmental awareness reduces stress and improves emotional regulation. Acceptance doesn't mean passivity—it's an active choice to meet life as it is, creating more space for clarity, compassion, and growth.

Daily activity

Release

Close your eyes and picture your hands curled into fists.
Imagine all the judgments you carry clenched there.
Now slowly open your hands—palms up, relaxed.
As you breathe, envision letting go of each one.
Feel the space that opens in their absence.

There's no perfect way to be present.
There's only this moment
and your willingness to meet it again and again.

Releasing Verdicts

What does it feel like to simply notice your thoughts without trying to change or label them?

Can you recall a moment when you didn't cling to or push away your thinking? When you let it pass through like weather? What did that feel like in your body?
Peaceful? Unfamiliar? Disorienting?
Let yourself return to that space now.
What happens when you allow thoughts without wrestling them?
Mindfulness practices rooted in cognitive neuroscience show that observing thoughts
—without reacting—
reduces reactivity in the brain's fear centers. This gentle witnessing builds resilience and calm, offering clarity without force.

Daily activity

"I am but an observer"

Find a quiet space.
Close your eyes and let your thoughts come and go.
Don't follow them or push them away.
Just label them softly:
"thinking," "remembering," "judging,"
then return to your breath.
No fixing. Just noticing.

Your thoughts are not you.
Let them pass like clouds, and feel the sky behind them widen.

Date: _____

Releasing Verdicts

What judgments do you hold about your mindfulness practice itself?

Do you ever feel like you're doing it "wrong"?
That it's too hard, too quiet, not deep enough?
Where did those expectations come from?
Someone else's definition of progress, or your own inner critic?
What might your practice feel like if you let go of how it should look, and met it simply as it is?
Research in contemplative psychology suggests that self-judgment during meditation can actually inhibit its benefits by activating stress pathways. But when we drop expectations and return to curiosity, the brain shifts into more relaxed, integrative states.

Daily activity

Gentle Return

During your next mindfulness session, every time you notice yourself judging the practice
"This isn't working," "I'm not focused"
pause.
Label the thought "judging."
Then softly return to your breath.
Each return is the practice.

Mindfulness isn't about stillness
It's about honesty.

Date: _____

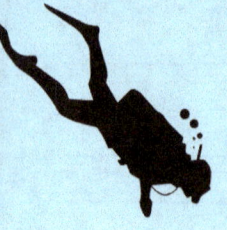

Take a moment. Really take it.

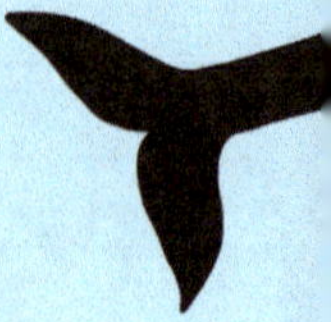

<u>You're doing it.</u>

It may not always be graceful.
The results may not be instant.
But you are showing up. Again and again.
You're putting in the work.
You're putting yourself first — even if it's just for these few
moments each day.
And that matters.
So pause. Breathe. Acknowledge just how far you've come.
That's seven more activities, check-ins, and journal entries under
your belt.
That's seven more times you chose you.
You have earned a break. A full, unapologetic, soul-soothing day of
rest.
Put the journal down for now and simply be.
You deserve that.

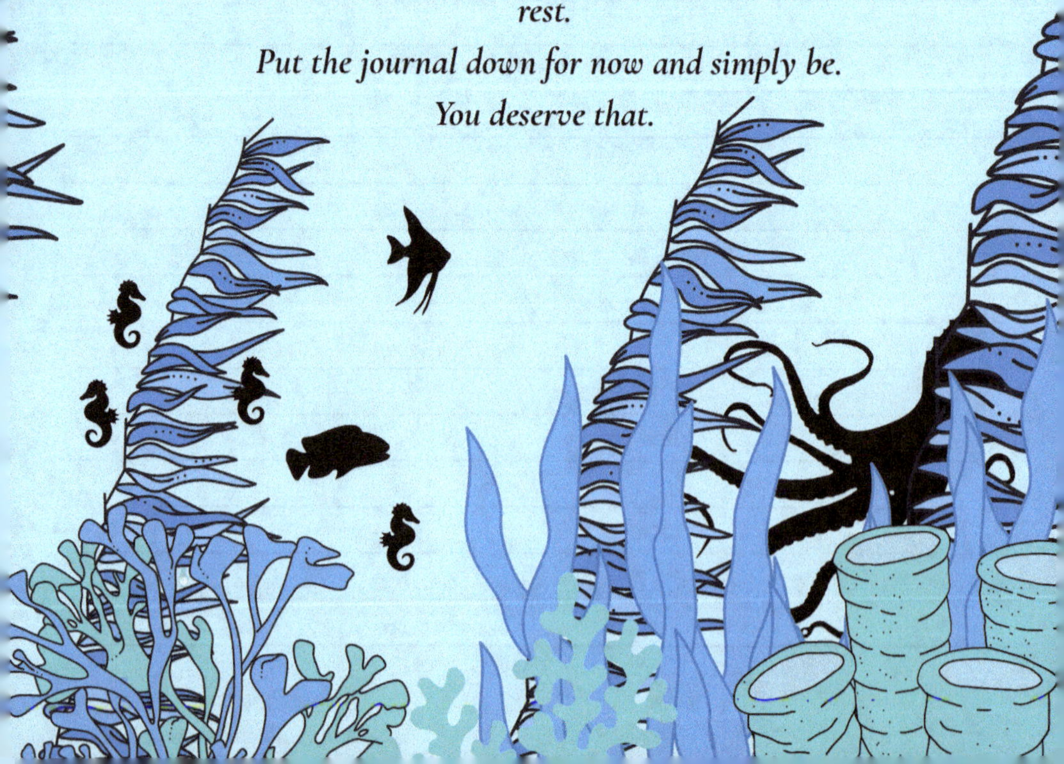

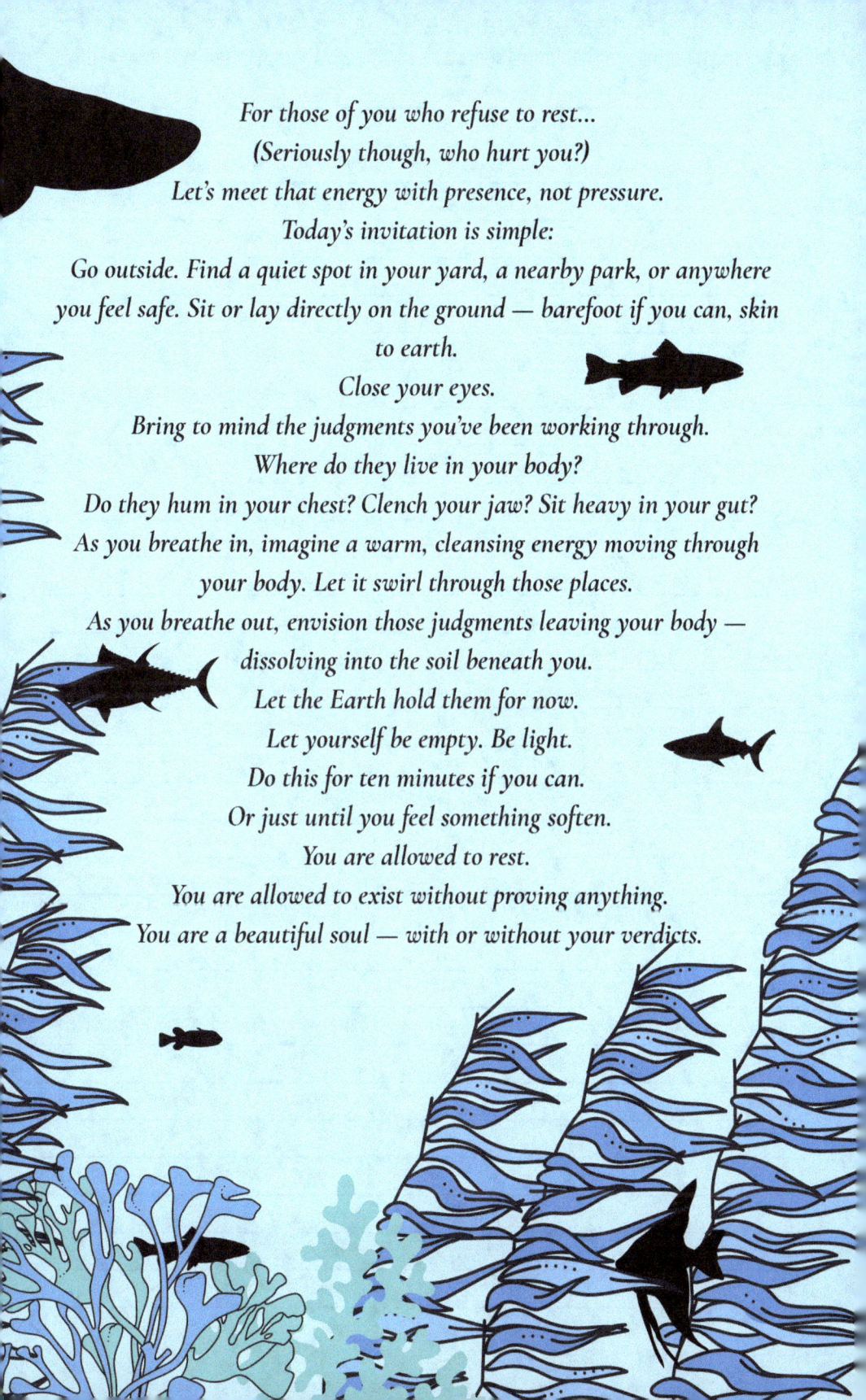

For those of you who refuse to rest...
(Seriously though, who hurt you?)
Let's meet that energy with presence, not pressure.
Today's invitation is simple:
Go outside. Find a quiet spot in your yard, a nearby park, or anywhere
you feel safe. Sit or lay directly on the ground — barefoot if you can, skin
to earth.
Close your eyes.
Bring to mind the judgments you've been working through.
Where do they live in your body?
Do they hum in your chest? Clench your jaw? Sit heavy in your gut?
As you breathe in, imagine a warm, cleansing energy moving through
your body. Let it swirl through those places.
As you breathe out, envision those judgments leaving your body —
dissolving into the soil beneath you.
Let the Earth hold them for now.
Let yourself be empty. Be light.
Do this for ten minutes if you can.
Or just until you feel something soften.
You are allowed to rest.
You are allowed to exist without proving anything.
You are a beautiful soul — with or without your verdicts.

Date: _____

Date: _____

Releasing Verdicts

Recall a time when releasing judgment brought you relief or clarity.

What shifted inside when you stopped needing to label a person, moment, or feeling as good or bad?
Did something soften?
Your breath, your shoulders, your heart?
Let yourself return to that space. What was different?
What became available when you let go?
Studies in mindfulness and affect regulation show that releasing judgment, even briefly, reduces activity in the brain's default mode network
—linked to rumination and stress—
and increases emotional flexibility. It creates space for insight to emerge naturally.

Daily activity

Anchored in Peace:

Sit in stillness and gently recall a moment when nonjudgment brought you peace.
Close your eyes and relive it through the senses.
Where were you? What were you feeling?
Let the memory anchor your body now.
Breathe it in, without needing to change a thing.

Relief doesn't always come from answers
Sometimes it comes from letting go.

Date: _____

Releasing Verdicts

How does comparing yourself to others feed judgment?

When you place yourself beside someone else
—on success, appearance, healing, or even peace—
what happens inside?
Do you shrink, strive, justify, or compete?
What judgments are born in that space, and whose standards
are you using?
Comparison activates regions of the brain tied to
self-evaluation and social ranking, which can heighten
insecurity, envy, or superiority. Mindfulness invites us to
interrupt that cycle and return to presence, where worth isn't
a contest.

Daily activity

I'm Enough

Each time you catch yourself comparing today, pause.
Place your hand on your chest and say gently,
"I am enough in this moment."
Then redirect your focus inward:
What am I learning? What do I need?
Let that guide you instead of the outside.

Comparison is a thief that wears your own face.

Date: _____

Releasing Verdicts

What if you met yourself today with the same patience you'd offer someone you love?

Where might that shift how you speak, move, decide, or rest?
What tone would your inner voice take?
What might soften in your body if you didn't rush to fix, scold, or perform?
Could you let mistakes or confusion simply exist?
Without punishment?
Studies show that self-compassion increases emotional resilience, reduces stress, and strengthens motivation. It isn't indulgence—it's alignment with how the nervous system heals and grows. Patience quiets the fear that we are only worthy when perfect.

Daily activity

Self Love's the Best Love

Stand or sit in front of a mirror.
Look into your own eyes and
with intention
say something kind as if to a dear friend:
"You're doing your best," or "I'm proud of you."
Repeat it gently, even if it feels awkward.
ESPECIALLY if it feels awkward.
Watch what shifts.

The love you offer others is not foreign to you, it lives within you.
All that's needed is permission to turn it inward.
Let today be that permission.

Date: _____

Releasing Verdicts

What does self-acceptance mean to you?

Is it peace with your past? Gentleness in the mirror? The
freedom to be unfinished?
Imagine what it would feel like to accept every part of yourself.
Not just the polished or productive bits.
What draws you toward that vision? What part of it still feels
hard to claim?
Psychology shows that self-acceptance is one of the
strongest predictors of well-being,
yet it's often the most neglected.
Unlike self-esteem, it's not about achievement
it's about unconditional presence.
Accepting yourself doesn't mean giving up.
It means starting from a place of wholeness instead of lack.

Daily activity

If I was my own friend

Write a short letter to yourself from the perspective of
someone who loves you unconditionally.
Acknowledge your struggles, your effort, your growth.
Let it be soft, honest, and kind.
Read it back slowly, like it matters.
Because it does.

Self-acceptance doesn't mean you stop growing
It means you stop shrinking to grow.

Date: _____

Releasing Verdicts

What labels do you habitually apply to yourself—like lazy, anxious, strong, weak, too much, not enough?

Where did these labels come from?
Were they whispered by family, stamped by systems, or forged in moments of pain? Which ones have you clung to?
Which ones were never really yours?
Explore how these words shape your choices, posture, self-worth—and whether you're ready to let any of them go.
Neuroscience shows that repeated self-labeling shapes neural pathways
Reinforcing both belief and behavior.
But what's wired can be rewired.
Awareness is the first interruption of the script.

Daily activity

Sacrificing Labels

Write down 1–3 labels you've carried that no longer serve you. Fold the paper, then:
Destroy it (safely),
Rip it up,
Or bury it under a stone.
As you do, silently say:
"I am not this name. I am something deeper."
Let the act be a quiet declaration of freedom

You are not the words the world gave you.
You are what rises in spite of them.

Date: _____

Releasing Verdicts

How do you respond when others judge you?

Do you shrink, defend, shut down, or pretend not to care?
Where in your body do you feel it first?
chest, gut, throat?
How much power do others' opinions hold over how you see
yourself and why?
Explore what shifts when you choose to stand in your truth,
even if you're misunderstood.
Social rejection activates the same brain regions as physical
pain. But resilience grows when we root our worth internally.
Not in the reactions of others.

Daily activity

Roots

Stand barefoot on the grass or ground.
Shift your weight side to side, then front to back.
Settle into stillness and press gently into the ground.
With each inhale, imagine drawing up your own strength.
With each exhale, release others' projections.
Let the ground remind you:
You are already whole.

You are not required to carry every opinion handed to you.

Releasing Verdicts

What are you afraid would happen if you stopped judging altogether?

Would you lose your edge? Be taken advantage of?
Feel lost or directionless?
Judgment often builds walls to feel safe or certain.
What does it protect you from?
Discomfort? Vulnerability? Chaos?
Explore what it would feel like to lower that shield, even briefly.
Would you be less protected?...
Or more free?
Research shows that the brain prefers predictable patterns,
even if they cause stress.
Judgment can act like scaffolding for the ego
but spacious awareness often brings greater clarity, not less.

Daily activity

This Too Shall Pass

Sit comfortably and rest your hands, palms up.
Inhale deeply and say silently:
"I don't need to judge this."
Exhale:
"I allow this moment."
Let openness in the hands signal openness in the mind.
Don't chase thoughts
Just notice.

You don't have to label the moment to live it.
Sometimes peace arrives when we let go of naming everything.

Date: _____

Good morning, afternoon, and evening,
Dear reader,
You've blasted through another 7 days of prompts
(not surprised—you're amazing)
You showed up again and again for you.
That's something most people never do.
So next time someone questions your discipline or
growth, remind them:
you're walking a path they don't even see.
If someone bribed you to do this—good on them. Getting
paid to grow? A dream. But whether you're here for
healing, discovery, or curiosity, you've earned this rest.
And even if you hadn't, you still deserve it.

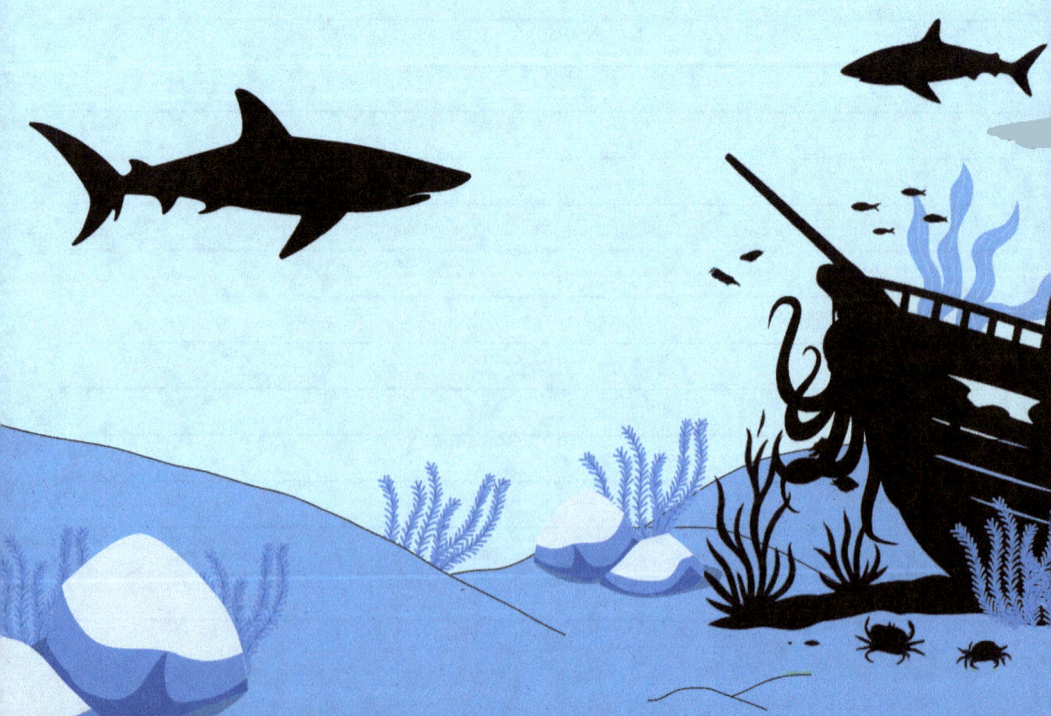

For the ones who can't sit still
(you know who you are):

Face Yourself – A Mirror Practice

Find a quiet space with a mirror and soft
lighting (bathroom mirror is fine).
Sit or stand. Look into your own eyes for at
least 2 minutes. <u>Let it be uncomfortable.</u>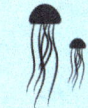
Notice the judgments that arise.
Ask: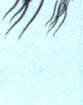
Is this true, or something I was told to believe?
Write them down.
Then rewrite each with compassion.
Example: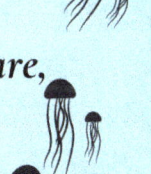
"You look tired." → "My body is asking for care,
not criticism."
End by gently washing your face.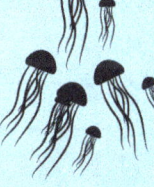
Release what isn't yours.

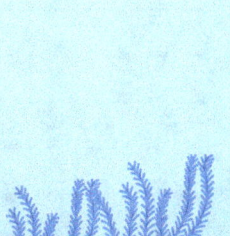

Date: _____

Date: _____

Releasing Verdicts

What role does judgment play in your sense of control?

Do you judge to stay one step ahead? To avoid risk? To feel certainty in uncertainty?
Judgment often acts as a shield against chaos
it gives structure to the unknown. But does that control bring ease... or tension? Explore whether judgment helps you feel safe, or simply in charge. What might soften if you allowed life to unfold without needing to manage every angle? Neuroscience suggests the brain is wired to predict, and judgment is one way it tries to impose order. Yet over-controlling can increase anxiety, not reduce it. Letting go activates the parasympathetic nervous system—your body's natural calm.

Daily activity

Letting Go

Choose one area of your life where you feel the need to stay in control. For just a few minutes today, consciously release that grip:
Let the house be a little messy.
Let someone else lead.
Let yourself not know.
As you do, silently repeat:
"I don't need to judge this to be with it."
Observe what softens—and what resists.

True strength isn't always found in control
It often lives in your willingness to let go

Date: _____

Releasing Verdicts

When you combine Beginner's Mind with Non-Judging, how does that change your perception of judgment?

Does it feel softer? More human? Less absolute? Beginner's Mind says I don't know yet. Non-Judging says and that's okay. Together, they offer a powerful pause—a way to witness your inner world without rushing to conclusions. What happens when you meet your judgments with curiosity instead of resistance—when you let questions replace answers? What new space opens up inside you when you're allowed to not know and not label at the same time? Psychology calls this "decentering"—the ability to observe thoughts and judgments without fusing with them. It's linked to greater emotional resilience, creativity, and reduced anxiety. Wonder and acceptance, when combined, create fertile ground for transformation.

Daily activity

Is that the whole story?

Choose one judgmental thought you've had today. Write it down. Then ask yourself: "What else could be true here?" or "What haven't I considered?" Gently reframe the thought through the lens of curiosity instead of critique. Let your mind wander, wonder, and expand.

When judgment meets wonder, the edges soften.
You are allowed to not know.
You are allowed to be kind in your not-knowing.

Date: _____

Releasing Verdicts

When do you notice judgment arise most automatically? Toward yourself or others?

What moments trigger it without your conscious awareness? Do you catch yourself mid-thought, or only after it's already shaped your mood or action? Maybe you dont catch it until you sit and actively look for it? Explore what patterns you find, and ask yourself: how would it feel to simply witness the judgment arise, rather than obey it?

We all carry mental shortcuts

Biases that fire before we've even noticed.

Neuroscience calls them "default mode" reactions, formed by repetition and reinforced by emotion. But awareness interrupts the automatic. The act of noticing gives you space to choose a different response.

Non-judging isn't about silencing the voice

It's about learning not to take orders from it.

Daily activity

The 3-Breath Check-In

Set an intention to pause whenever you feel tension, irritation, or self-doubt.
Close your eyes and take three slow, conscious breaths.
With each inhale, notice what's rising.
With each exhale, release any need to label it.
This micro-moment of awareness can shift the course of your day.

Judgment often consumes more energy than acceptance.

Releasing Verdicts

How does judging yourself or others drain your energy?

Notice how quickly judgment tightens the body, clouds the mind, or pulls you out of the present? What inner tension does it create? How much effort goes into maintaining your evaluations?
trying to be right, stay guarded, or avoid feeling?
What might be possible with that energy freed up?
Judgment isn't passive
It consumes mental bandwidth, triggers stress responses, and contracts your attention. Studies show that negative self-talk activates the brain's threat circuitry, raising cortisol and keeping the nervous system in subtle defense. Every judgment is a story you must uphold—consciously or not. And stories take energy. What could you create with that power reclaimed?

Daily activity

Thought softener

Spend 10–15 minutes in free, intuitive movement
Stretching, shaking, dancing, or even rolling on the floor.
As you move, imagine releasing each judgment you've held today, letting it fall from your body like water off your skin.
Let movement soften where thoughts have hardened.

Judgment holds tight. Presence opens.
Let the energy that once fueled self-defense fuel your freedom instead.

Date: _____

Releasing Verdicts

What judgments do you still hold about your past self?

About decisions made, paths taken, things you said or didn't say? Imagine that version of you not as a failure, but as someone doing the best they could with what they knew. What would it feel like to finally make peace with them? Neuroscience reminds us that the brain is constantly rewiring itself so what feels obvious now may have been inaccessible then. Shame and regret often arise when we apply today's awareness to yesterday's choices.
But
your past self wasn't lesser
they were simply in process.
Acceptance doesn't mean approval
it means recognizing the humanity in who you were.
The work is not to rewrite the past, but to unhook from the judgment that keeps you bound to it.

Daily activity

Dear me

Take 10–15 minutes to write a compassionate letter to a former version of yourself.
Address their fears, celebrate their courage, and forgive their missteps.
Let your current self be the voice of grace they didn't yet know how to offer.

Peace isn't found by changing the past
Only by softening toward it. You grew from it. That counts.

Date: _____

Releasing Verdicts

What do you believe you must "fix" about yourself before you can be at peace?

Is there a part of you you've placed on hold?
some trait, flaw, or habit you feel must be corrected before you deserve rest, love, or acceptance?
Where did that belief come from?
What if peace didn't come after healing... but made healing possible?
Many of us internalize the belief that worth must be earned through improvement. But research in self-compassion and trauma recovery shows the opposite:
healing deepens when we feel safe and accepted,
not when we feel broken.
Inner change rarely grows from shame.
It grows from being seen and met where we are.
You don't have to be "better" to be whole.
Sometimes, the act of letting go of the fixing is what lets the healing begin.

Daily activity

Mirror Reflection (Compassion Gaze)

Stand before a mirror and look into your own eyes for 60 seconds. As you do, breathe slowly and say inwardly, "There is nothing I must fix before I can rest." Repeat a few times. Notice any resistance—and stay with it gently. You're learning to meet yourself with kindness, not critique.

Peace isn't the prize for perfection.
It's the ground from which transformation can finally bloom.

Date: _____

Releasing Verdicts

How does judging others create distance between you?

Think of a time when judgment formed a wall between you and someone else. What assumptions did you make about their worth, motives, or character? How did it change your body language, tone, or willingness to listen?
What do you think was lost in that moment—connection, understanding, ease? What might have been different if curiosity had come first?
Social neuroscience shows that when we judge others, we activate the brain's self-protection systems—literally narrowing our perception and reducing empathy. This makes it harder to see nuance, to listen fully, or to hold space for someone else's complexity. Curiosity, on the other hand, opens us—widening attention, softening defenses, and inviting presence. Connection doesn't require agreement, but it does ask for openness.

Daily activity

Curiosity Reframe Exercise

Choose one person you've judged recently, even subtly. Today, write down three genuine questions about them you don't know the answer to—things that, if explored, might build understanding. You don't need to ask them out loud—just practice replacing assumption with inquiry.

Judgment builds walls. Curiosity builds bridges.
Which do you want between you?

Date: _____

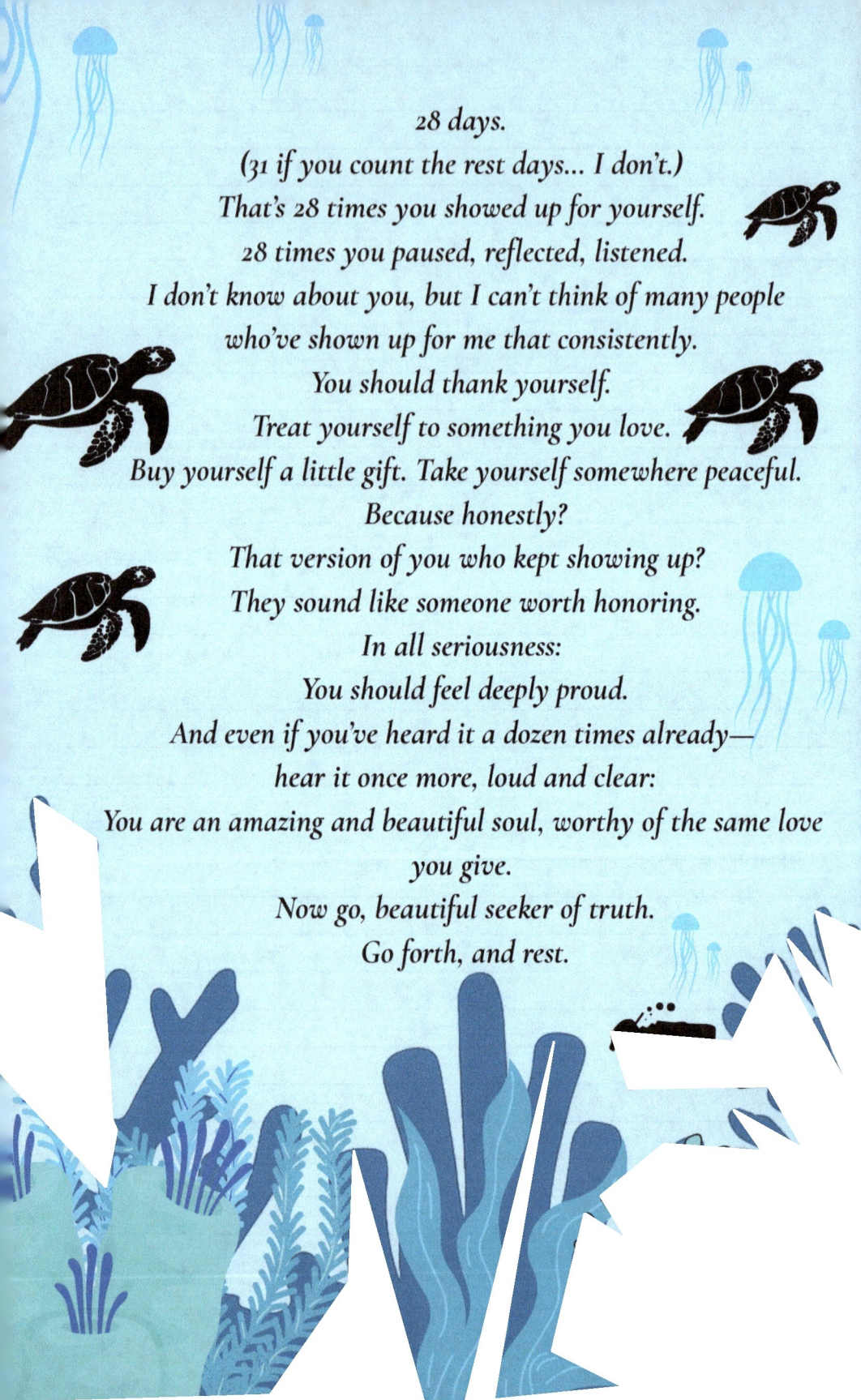

28 days.
(31 if you count the rest days... I don't.)
That's 28 times you showed up for yourself.
28 times you paused, reflected, listened.
I don't know about you, but I can't think of many people
who've shown up for me that consistently.
You should thank yourself.
Treat yourself to something you love.
Buy yourself a little gift. Take yourself somewhere peaceful.
Because honestly?
That version of you who kept showing up?
They sound like someone worth honoring.
In all seriousness:
You should feel deeply proud.
And even if you've heard it a dozen times already—
hear it once more, loud and clear:
You are an amazing and beautiful soul, worthy of the same love
you give.
Now go, beautiful seeker of truth.
Go forth, and rest.

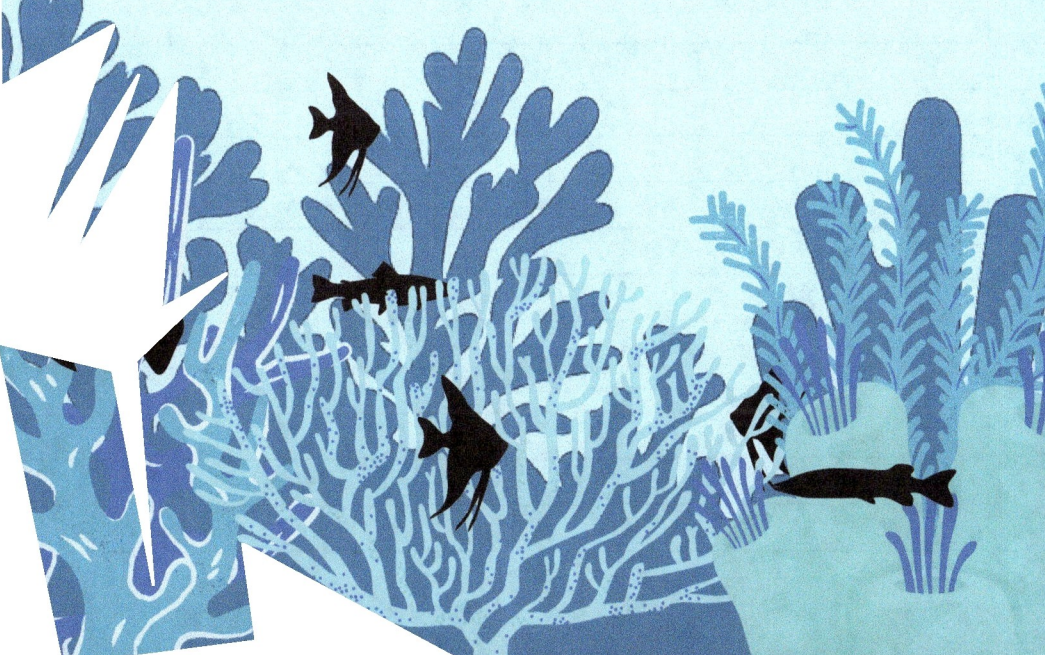

Hello again, my dear relentless workaholic.
I know you're here looking for one last invitation to do.
Fine. I've got you.
Today's practice is this:
Find a space where you can sit or lay down for ten full minutes.
Set a timer.
Get comfortable.
Now here comes the tricky part...
Do nothing.
Seriously.
No journaling. No planning. No problem-solving.
Just exist. For ten minutes.
No verdicts. No fixing. No effort.
When your timer goes off, give yourself a high five.
A gentle pat.
Or if you're feeling bold... smack your bottom and say:
"Good [insert your pronoun here]."
Because you are.
I love you.
But seriously—learn to rest without needing permission.

Date: _____

Date: _____

Releasing Verdicts

Why do you think it's okay to judge?
Why do you think it's wrong?

Judgment is rarely just about the moment
It's a pattern built from past pain, cultural conditioning, and internalized fear. Sometimes it feels like power. Sometimes it feels like safety. But often, it's a reflex that keeps us from truly seeing what's in front of us.
From a psychological lens, judgment can offer temporary certainty but at the cost of connection.
Somatically, you might feel it tighten your jaw, your chest, your gut—body bracing against discomfort.
Spiritually, it may pull you further from compassion, both for others and yourself.
What part of you feels protected by judgment? What part longs to be free from it? Can you sit in that space without rushing to label one side as right?

Daily activity

Their Shoes
Choose one person you've recently judged.
Write a short paragraph from their imagined perspective.
What might they be feeling, fearing, or trying to protect?
This practice activates the brain's medial prefrontal cortex—linked to empathy and social understanding and helps interrupt black-and-white thinking.
Let yourself feel their humanity, even if you still disagree.

Sometimes judgment is a shield we raise
When understanding feels too vulnerable.

Date: _____

Releasing Verdicts

How do you judge your progress in mindfulness?

Do you expect to feel calmer? Think less? Be perfect at "doing it right"?

If you've ever felt like you were failing at presence, ask yourself: whose voice is measuring that failure? Is it your own, or one you inherited?

Psychologically, we're wired to seek progress we can see—but mindfulness unfolds in subtler ways. Sometimes "progress" is simply noticing when you're lost in thought. Sometimes it's catching yourself judging—and choosing not to follow that trail.

Spiritually, mindfulness is not about arrival—it's about returning.

Again.

And again.

What if being "off-track" is part of the track?

Daily activity

Proof-Reading Self

Set a soft chime or vibration to go off randomly 2–3 times today. When it sounds, pause and ask:

"What story am I telling myself right now?"

No fixing—just noticing.

This practice builds metacognitive awareness, gently rewiring the brain toward non-reactivity.

You are not behind. You're not doing it wrong.
Every time you notice you've wandered off...
that's the practice. That's the miracle.

Releasing Verdicts

Looking back over the past 30 days, how has your relationship to judgment changed?

What have you learned about yourself—your habits, your softness, your strength? Have you found moments where you observed your mind instead of reacting? Where compassion replaced critique?
Neuroscience shows that nonjudging awareness quiets emotional reactivity and strengthens regulation. But even deeper is the felt sense
When tension softens, breath slows, and space opens within. You are not your thoughts. You never were. What surprised you this month? What shifted? What are you proud of—and what part of this gentler awareness will you carry forward?

Daily activity

Integration Walk

Take a slow walk
inside or outside
With the intention of reviewing your journey.
Each step, each breath, a moment of reflection.
Don't force insights. Simply invite them.
Let your body remember what your mind may have missed.
At the end of your walk, pause... and offer yourself this silent phrase:
"I can meet this moment just as I am."

You are not who you were 30 days ago.
You're the one who showed up.

Date: _____

Date: _____

Date: _____

Dear reader,

Congratulations on completing—or even just considering—this 30-day journey.

Whether you showed up each day in perfect rhythm or touched down here and there when you could, the truth remains:

you showed up for yourself.

That matters.

In a world constantly pulling us outward, you paused.

You reflected.

You gave yourself space to be.

You may have skipped pages, circled back, or barely started.

That's okay.

Even reading this now is a form of presence.

A moment of choosing you.

It is our sincerest wish here at LostBreeze that something within these pages stirred something in you

a thought, a truth, a shift.

Even the smallest spark can light the way forward.

If you'd like to stay connected or share your experience, we'd love to hear from you.

Join the conversation on Instagram or Facebook—scan the code at the back of this journal.

Your story might be just what someone else needs to hear.

Until then,

Keep breathing.

Keep returning.

You're doing better than you think.

With warmth,

—The LostBreeze Team

Mindfulness isn't a one-time achievement. It's a way of meeting yourself—again and again—with curiosity and care.

Why it matters

Psychologically:

Studies on mindfulness-based practices show consistent benefits for mood regulation, attention, and stress reduction. Just 10–15 minutes of mindful reflection per day can lower cortisol, improve sleep, and increase gray matter in areas linked to emotional awareness and compassion.

What to watch for Somatically:

As you move through life, begin to notice:

Tension in your jaw or shoulders?

Shallow breathing?

A tendency to "bristle" or shut down?

These are physical cues of judgment and emotional overload.

Mindfulness helps decode them before they take root.

Try these simple resets:

Neck rolls and shoulder shrugs to release tension

Legs up the wall pose (Viparita Karani) to calm the nervous system

Box breathing (4–4–4–4) to ground during anxious moments

Place your hand on your heart and say: "I am here. I am enough."

Spiritually speaking:

Mindfulness returns you to the sacred ordinary—the hum of breath, the feel of sunlight, the kindness in your own gaze.

Don't strive for perfect peace. Just return to you. That's the path.

That's the practice.

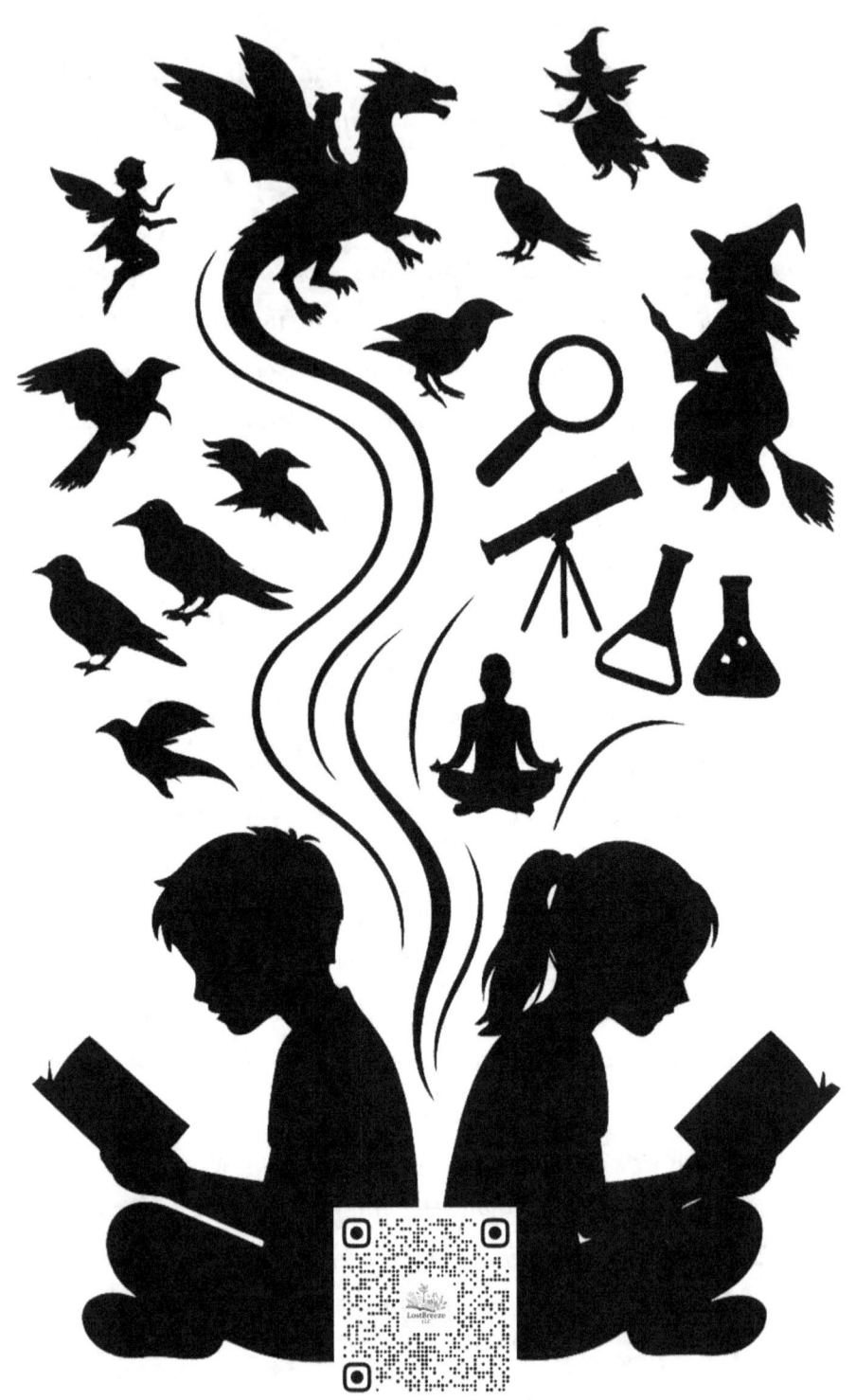

www.ingramcontent.com/pod-product-compliance
Lightning Source LLC
Chambersburg PA
CBHW070642130626
46555CB00006B/2658